Inhaling Freedom

Unlocking the Power of Conscious Breathing

By

Dr. Robert J. Coleman

Table of contents

Introduction:

Welcome to "Inhaling Freedom" an ebook that will change your perspective on the breath and its significant impact on your general well-being. In this digital guide, we will go on a trip to discover the remarkable power of mindful breathing, revealing how it may improve physical health, mental clarity, and emotional balance.

Breathing is an automatic action that has been with us since the moment we were born. However, how often do we pause to ponder the true power and potential that each breath contains? The Breathable Body seeks to illuminate the art of conscious breathing by presenting ideas, techniques, and practical exercises that can transform how you perceive and participate with your breath.
Various civilizations and traditions have acknowledged the value of breath as a portal to self-discovery and transformation throughout history. Breathwork has been used to nurture inner calm, promote healing, and extend consciousness throughout history, from ancient yogic techniques to

mindfulness meditation. This ebook presents a full investigation of breathwork, presenting it as a vital tool for personal growth and self-care in the modern world, drawing on these old wisdom traditions as well as contemporary scientific studies.
The book "The Breathable Body" is divided into sections, each of which focuses on a distinct component of conscious breathing. We'll look at the physiological mechanisms of breathing and how they affect our nervous system, cardiovascular health, and immune response. Furthermore, we will investigate the significant links between breath and cognition, studying how mindful breathing can reduce stress, improve focus, and promote emotional well-being.

This booklet will walk you through a series of practical activities meant to increase your understanding and experience of aware breathing, in addition to theoretical explanations. You will learn a variety of breathwork techniques, such as diaphragmatic breathing, alternate nostril breathing, and rhythmic breathing. These practices are simple to adopt into your everyday routine, allowing you to tap into the transforming power of each breath. Whether you want to reduce worry, increase your energy, or simply improve your overall quality of life, "The Breathable Body" is your entire guide to mindful breathing. You will embark on a wonderful journey of self-discovery, resilience, and empowerment by tapping into the innate wisdom of your breath.

Prepare to go on an astonishing journey into the realm of the breath, and discover how your breath holds the secret to realizing your full potential in body, mind, and spirit. Allow "The Breathable Body" to accompany you on your transformational journey of conscious living.

Chapter.1

Your Nose Has the Potential to Save Your Life

The human body is a remarkable machine that is precisely designed to protect and sustain itself. Over millions of years, it has developed to adapt to its surroundings, living and thriving in a variety of conditions. The nose is one of our bodies' most astounding features, an organ that is often overlooked despite its incredible ability to detect and analyze scents. In this book, we will delve into the fascinating world of the "breathable body" and discover the olfactory system's secret powers. Consider a world without the ability to smell. It would be a life without color, without the vivid tapestry of smells that shapes our view of the world. The smell is frequently associated with positive experiences, such as the aroma of freshly baked bread, the lovely perfume of blooming flowers, or the soothing fragrance of a loved one. However, the full power of our sense of smell extends beyond simply pleasure. It is crucial to our survival.

Have you ever gone into a room and knew something was amiss before your eyes even recognized any outward signs? It may have been the subtle stench of gas leaking from a broken stove or the harsh odor of burnt wiring. Your nose served as a silent sentinel, alerting you to impending danger. Our olfactory system is intended to serve as an early warning system, capable of detecting the presence of harmful compounds, diseases, or even imminent therapy situations.

Consider Sarah, a young woman who narrowly avoided a house fire due to her excellent sense of smell. A defective electrical line sparked in the walls while she slept comfortably one fatal night. The house began to fill with smoke, as deadly carbon monoxide gas spread stealthily across the rooms. Sarah was startled awake by the odor of burning plastic and quickly covered her nose and mouth with a damp cloth. She navigated the smoke-filled halls using her olfactory capabilities and managed to escape before the fire engulfed the entire building.

Sarah's experience is not an isolated one. The extraordinary power of our noses has saved countless lives. Our olfactory system acts as a dedicated protector, continuously working to keep us safe, from detecting bad food to recognizing harmful compounds. However, in a world dominated by visual cues, we frequently ignore the value of our sense of smell. It is time to recognize and exploit this untapped superpower.

In the next chapters, we shall delve deeply into the olfactory system's complicated workings. We'll look at the architecture of the nose, the sophisticated network of sensors, and how the brain processes scent information. We will discover how various fragrances influence our emotions, memories, and overall well-being. Furthermore, we will learn how to improve and train our sense of smell, allowing us to live a better and safer life.

So, join me on this exciting voyage into the world of "Inhaling Freedom:" and find the untapped potential just under our eyes. We will discover secrets that will save lives, enrich experiences, and remind us of the astounding intricacy of the human body. Remember that your nose can save your life.

Chapter 2

Unleash the Scented Symphony

As we continue our exploration of the human nose, we enter a realm of delicate scents and scented symphonies. The nose not only has the incredible ability to detect a vast range of aromas, but it also has the ability to transport us to distant memories and elicit strong emotions. Inhaling freedom, we dig further into this sensory masterpiece's unique anatomy.

A sophisticated network of olfactory sensors awaits its next encounter with the fragrant universe within the nasal cavity. These unique cells found deep within the nasal epithelium, have an incredible ability to capture the essence of our surroundings. aroma molecules move through the air as we breathe in, creating their own aroma way to the olfactory receptors, which are waiting for them.

Consider this: you're strolling through a gorgeous garden filled with vibrant flowers of all colors. The gentle breeze transports the beautiful fragrances of blooming roses, freshly cut grass, and fragrant honeysuckle, while the warm sun caresses your skin. The air flows through your nasal passages with each breath, triggering a symphony of scents within your sensory system.

When scent molecules reach the olfactory receptors, they bind to certain proteins, beginning a chain reaction of metabolic reactions. These complex impulses are sent to the olfactory bulb, a structure at the base of the brain where the magic truly begins. The signals are converted here into electrical impulses that go via the olfactory nerve to the olfactory cortex.

The full power of fragrance is unleashed in the olfactory cortex, which is delicately linked throughout the brain's huge neuronal network. This area is in charge of processing and interpreting olfactory bulb information and converting them into meaningful impressions. Memories, emotions, and associations associated with specific fragrances are created inside these brain circuits.

Consider the captivating allure of freshly baked bread, permeating a warm and inviting kitchen. As its tantalizing aroma drifts through the air, it delicately caresses the olfactory receptors nestled within our noses, setting off a symphony of neural activity. Instantaneously, a flood of cherished memories, infused with the comforting scent, rushes through our minds, invoking vivid images of a grandmother's loving embrace. The fragrance serves as a time machine, transporting us to moments that hold profound significance, serving as a sensory portal to the past.

Beyond its capacity to evoke memories, the olfactory cortex possesses the remarkable ability to awaken deep-rooted emotions within us. The scent of a fragrant pine forest may elicit a sense of tranquility and inner peace, whereas the acrid odor of smoke may arouse feelings of fear and caution. Whether it be the sweet fragrance of a lover's perfume or the nostalgic scent of a childhood home, the olfactory cortex intricately weaves a tapestry of emotions, imbuing our experiences with vivid hues.

Yet, the journey of scent does not cease there. Our sense of smell works in tandem with our sense of taste, creating a multisensory experience that enriches our perception of flavors. When we relish a delectable meal, the olfactory receptors in our nose play a vital role in detecting the intricate aromas that contribute to the overall flavor profile. It is no wonder that a congested nose, stifling our ability to detect scents, diminishes our enjoyment of food.

As we delve deeper into the intricate anatomy of the nose, we discover the extraordinary power it holds. Beyond its biological function of detecting odors, the nose serves as a gateway to our memories, emotions, and the world that surrounds us. It beckons us to revel in the symphony of scents that envelops our existence, reminding us of the intricate beauty and profound complexity of the human experience.

Let us now explore the fundamental aspects of the olfactory system, the very foundation of our sense of smell, with a closer lens:

The journey of the olfactory system commences with specialized sensory receptors known as olfactory receptor neurons (ORNs). These remarkable receptors reside within the olfactory epithelium, a minuscule patch of tissue located high inside the nasal cavity. Equipped with specialized receptor proteins on their surface, ORNs possess the ability to detect a diverse array of odor molecules present in the surrounding environment.

1. Odorant Molecules: Fragrant molecules, referred to as odorants, are volatile chemicals that emanate from various objects and substances around us. When we inhale, some of these odorants enter our nasal cavity and come into contact with the olfactory epithelium.

2. Olfactory Epithelium: Nestled within the olfactory epithelium reside millions of olfactory receptor neurons, each expressing a distinct type of olfactory receptor protein. These receptor proteins endow ORNs with the capacity to detect and bind to specific odorant molecules, initiating the olfactory journey.

3. Signal Transduction: When an odorant molecule binds to its corresponding receptor protein on an olfactory receptor neuron, a cascade of biochemical events is set into motion within the neuron. This intricate process, known as signal transduction, culminates in the generation of electrical signals called action potentials.

4. Olfactory Bulb: The action potentials generated by the olfactory receptor neurons embark on a remarkable voyage, traversing along bundled axons that collectively form the olfactory nerve. These nerve fibers project into the olfactory bulb, a specialized structure situated at the base of the brain.

5. Olfactory Cortex: The olfactory bulb serves as a relay station where sensory information is meticulously processed and subsequently transmitted
 to higher brain regions. From the olfactory bulb, signals are dispatched to the olfactory cortex, a region of the brain responsible for the intricate and nuanced processing of olfactory stimuli.

6. Brain Processing: The olfactory cortex establishes a network of connections with various other brain regions, including the amygdala, hippocampus, and frontal cortex. These intricate connections facilitate the integration of scent with memory, emotions, and cognitive processes, enabling us to recognize and respond to diverse odors.

7. Perception of Smell: Ultimately, the brain's complex processing of scent information culminates in the perception of smell. Different odorant molecules activate specific combinations of receptors, giving rise to the perception of various scents. Remarkably, the human brain possesses the ability to distinguish between thousands of distinct odors, affording us the capacity to identify and differentiate an astonishing range of smells.

The intricate network of sensors within the olfactory system, coupled with the awe-inspiring processing capabilities of the brain, endow us with the remarkable ability to perceive and interpret the world of smells. This sophisticated system plays an indispensable role in various facets of our lives, encompassing the appreciation of food, environmental awareness, and the richness of social interactions.

Chapter 3

Anatomy of breathing

The process of breathing is a fundamental physiological function that enables us to acquire the oxygen our bodies need while eliminating carbon dioxide, a waste product of cellular metabolism. It involves the intricate coordination of multiple structures and muscles within the respiratory system, ensuring the efficient exchange of gases. Let's delve further into the anatomy of breathing to gain a comprehensive understanding of this vital process:

1. Nasal Cavity: Breathing typically commences in the nasal cavity, where air enters the body through the nostrils. The nasal cavity acts as a crucial gateway, performing essential functions before the air reaches the lungs. Within this cavity, the air is filtered, moistened, and warmed to ensure optimal conditions for respiratory efficiency. Lining the nasal cavity are specialized structures called cilia, along with mucus-producing cells. These work together to trap and remove foreign particles, dust, and pathogens present in the inhaled air, thereby protecting the delicate respiratory system.

2. Pharynx: From the nasal cavity, the air proceeds to the pharynx, a muscular tube situated at the back of the throat. The pharynx serves as a common passageway for both air and food, performing the vital role of directing air toward the trachea during breathing. While swallowing, a mechanism called the epiglottis prevents food and liquids from entering the respiratory system by closing off the trachea.

3. Larynx: Located below the pharynx, the larynx, also known as the voice box, plays multiple roles in breathing. It contains the vocal cords, which are responsible for producing sound when air passes over them, allowing us to speak and produce various vocalizations. Moreover, the larynx acts as a protective mechanism by closing off during swallowing, effectively preventing food and liquid from entering the lower respiratory tract.

4. Trachea: Extending from the larynx into the chest, the trachea, often referred to as the windpipe, is a sturdy, flexible tube composed of cartilage rings. The trachea is lined with ciliated cells and goblet cells that produce mucus. The cilia, together with the mucus, efficiently trap inhaled particles and foreign substances, safeguarding the respiratory system from potential harm. Within the chest, the trachea divides into two narrower tubes known as the bronchi, which lead to the left and right lungs.

5. Bronchial Tree: Within the lungs, the bronchi continue to branch out, forming an intricate network of progressively smaller airways, aptly called the bronchial tree. As the bronchi divide further, they transform into smaller tubes called bronchioles, and this branching pattern continues until reaching the terminal bronchioles. The walls of the bronchial tree consist of smooth muscles and elastic connective tissue, enabling them to dilate or constrict, thereby regulating the airflow. This capability plays a crucial role in adapting to the varying respiratory demands of the body.

6. Alveoli: The terminal bronchioles culminate in clusters of microscopic air sacs called alveoli. These delicate structures are the primary sites of gas exchange within the lungs. The alveoli are encompassed by an intricate network of tiny blood vessels called capillaries. During inhalation, oxygen from the inhaled air effortlessly diffuses across the thin walls of the alveoli into the surrounding capillaries. Simultaneously, carbon dioxide, a waste product of cellular metabolism, moves from the capillaries into the alveoli to be expelled during exhalation.

7. Diaphragm and Intercostal Muscles: Integral to the process of breathing are two sets of muscles: the diaphragm and the intercostal muscles. The diaphragm, a dome-shaped muscle situated at the base of the chest cavity, plays a primary role in respiration. When it contracts and flattens, it creates more space within the chest cavity, leading to inhalation. Conversely, during exhalation, the diaphragm relaxes, while the intercostal muscles, located between the ribs, contract, causing the chest cavity volume to decrease. These coordinated actions facilitate the expulsion of air from the lungs.

8. Respiratory Centers: The intricate orchestration of breathing is regulated by specialized regions within the brainstem known as the respiratory centers. The primary respiratory center is the medulla oblongata, responsible for generating rhythmic signals that coordinate the contraction and relaxation of the respiratory muscles. These signals adjust the rate and depth of breathing in response to various factors, including the levels of carbon dioxide, oxygen, and pH in the blood. By continuously monitoring these variables, the respiratory centers ensure that the body's respiratory needs are met and maintained.

breathing encompasses the synchronized efforts of numerous structures, including the nasal cavity, pharynx, larynx, trachea, bronchial tree, alveoli, diaphragm, intercostal muscles, and the respiratory centers within the brainstem. This intricate and complex process enables the exchange of oxygen and carbon dioxide, providing the necessary support for the body's metabolic functions and overall well-being.

Chapter.4

Postures that support breathing

There are several postures that can support healthy breathing and improve lung capacity. By adopting these positions and practicing conscious breathing, you can optimize your respiratory function and enhance your overall well-being. Let's explore each posture in more detail:

1. Standing tall: Stand with your feet shoulder-width apart, your spine straight, and your shoulders relaxed. This posture allows for proper alignment of the respiratory system, enabling the lungs to expand fully. By maintaining an upright position, you create more space for your diaphragm to move efficiently and facilitate deep breathing.

2. Sitting upright: When sitting, ensure that your back is straight and your shoulders are relaxed. Avoid slouching or hunching over, as it can compress the chest and restrict breathing. By sitting upright, you maintain an open posture that supports optimal lung capacity and encourages efficient airflow.

3. Mountain pose (Tadasana): This foundational yoga posture involves standing with your feet together, spine straight, and arms relaxed at your sides. In Tadasana, you focus on grounding through your feet while elongating your spine and lifting the crown of your head. This alignment opens up the chest and encourages deep, diaphragmatic breathing, allowing the lungs to fully expand and increasing lung capacity.

4. Corpse pose (Savasana): Savasana is a relaxation posture in yoga that involves lying flat on your back with your arms at your sides and your legs slightly apart. It allows for unrestricted breathing and promotes a state of deep relaxation. By surrendering to the floor and consciously focusing on your breath, you can deepen your breath awareness and encourage fuller, more expansive breaths.

5. Forward folds: Forward bending poses, such as Uttanasana (standing forward bend) or

Paschimottanasana (seated forward bend), can help expand the back of the body and promote deeper breathing. These poses stretch the muscles of the back and create space in the chest, allowing for increased lung capacity and improved respiratory function.

6. Supported fish pose: Lie on your back with a yoga block or bolster placed horizontally under your upper back, just below the shoulder blades. This gentle backbend opens up the chest, stretches the front of the body, and facilitates fuller breaths. By providing support to the upper back, this pose encourages deep inhalations, allowing the lungs to expand more freely and enhancing breathing capacity.

7. Child's pose (Balasana): Kneel on the floor, bring your big toes together, and sit back on your heels. Lower your torso forward and rest it on your thighs, extending your arms forward or alongside your body. The child's pose promotes relaxation, deepens breath awareness, and allows for gentle expansion of the back and ribcage. By consciously breathing into your back body, you can improve the flexibility of your ribcage and enhance your overall breathing capacity.

In addition to practicing these postures, it is crucial to focus on slow, deep breathing and engage the diaphragm. Breathing deeply into the belly and filling the lungs completely ensures that you take in an ample oxygen supply and effectively release carbon dioxide. By combining good posture with conscious, deep breathing, you can optimize your respiratory function, increase lung capacity, and promote overall well-being.

Chapter.5

Buteyko of breathing education

The Buteyko Method, developed by Russian physician Konstantin Buteyko in the 1950s, is a breathing technique and educational program aimed at correcting dysfunctional breathing patterns and enhancing the body's tolerance to carbon dioxide (CO2) by reducing excessive breathing.

The fundamental principle of the Buteyko Method revolves around the notion that many individuals engage in over breathing, meaning they inhale more air than their bodies actually require. This habit can lead to various health issues, including asthma, anxiety, allergies, and sleep apnea. By retraining the breathing pattern to decrease the volume of the air intake, the Buteyko Method endeavors to restore normal breathing and promote overall well-being.

The Buteyko Method incorporates several key principles to achieve its objectives:

1. Nasal Breathing: The method emphasizes the importance of breathing through the nose rather than the mouth. The nose acts as a natural filter, humidifier, and regulator of air intake, optimizing the breathing process.

2. Reduced Breathing: The Buteyko Method encourages individuals to adopt slower, lighter, and more controlled breathing patterns. By maintaining a slightly reduced respiratory rate, it aims to enhance breathing efficiency.

3. Breath Holding: Short periods of breath holding are integrated into the Buteyko Method to increase the body's tolerance to higher levels of CO_2. This practice helps normalize breathing and trains the body to adapt to different oxygen and carbon dioxide levels.

4. Relaxation and Posture: The Buteyko Method places emphasis on relaxation techniques and correct posture. These factors contribute to the optimization of breathing efficiency and support overall respiratory function.

The Buteyko Method is commonly taught through individual or group sessions led by qualified instructors. Participants are guided through a series of exercises and techniques designed to retrain their breathing patterns. The program typically includes education about the physiological and biochemical aspects of breathing, as well as practical exercises aimed at gradually reducing breathing volume. Advocates of the Buteyko Method claim that it can yield various benefits, including improved respiratory function, alleviation of asthma symptoms, enhanced sleep quality, increased energy levels, and overall improved well-being. However, it is important to note that while some studies suggest positive outcomes, further high-quality research is needed to establish the effectiveness and long-term effects of the Buteyko Method.

If you are considering trying the Buteyko Method or have specific health concerns, it is strongly recommended to consult with a healthcare professional or a qualified Buteyko instructor. These experts can provide personalized guidance, and support, and address any individual considerations or needs.

Chapter.6

Dysfunctional breathing

Dysfunctional breathing, also known as disordered breathing or breathing pattern disorders, refers to an abnormal or inefficient way of breathing that can have a negative impact on a person's overall well-being and respiratory function. Breathing is an involuntary process essential for sustaining life, but when dysfunctional, it disrupts the natural, rhythmic pattern of breathing, leading to various physical and psychological symptoms.

Normal breathing involves the diaphragm, a dome-shaped muscle below the lungs, contracting and relaxing to facilitate the exchange of oxygen and carbon dioxide. The movement of the diaphragm creates a vacuum effect, causing the lungs to expand during inhalation and contract during exhalation. This type of breathing, known as diaphragmatic breathing or belly breathing, is considered the most efficient and natural.

On the other hand, dysfunctional breathing involves altered breathing patterns, such as shallow or rapid breathing, chest breathing (using the upper chest and shoulders instead of the diaphragm), or unintentionally holding the breath. These abnormal patterns disrupt the balance of oxygen and carbon dioxide in the body, impairing the efficiency of the respiratory system.

Several factors can contribute to the development of dysfunctional breathing. Psychological factors like stress, anxiety, and emotional trauma can lead to shallow or rapid breathing as a response to perceived threats or heightened arousal. Poor posture, a sedentary lifestyle, and chronic respiratory conditions like asthma or chronic obstructive pulmonary disease (COPD) can also contribute to dysfunctional breathing patterns.

The symptoms of dysfunctional breathing can vary widely and may manifest physically and psychologically. Common physical symptoms include shortness of breath, chest pain or discomfort, fatigue, dizziness, frequent sighing or yawning, and tightness in the chest or throat.

Psychological symptoms may include anxiety, panic attacks, poor concentration, irritability, and disrupted sleep patterns.

Dysfunctional breathing can have far-reaching consequences and affect multiple aspects of a person's health. Inefficient breathing patterns can lead to decreased oxygen delivery to the body's tissues and organs, resulting in fatigue, decreased exercise tolerance, and impaired cognitive function. Imbalanced levels of oxygen and carbon dioxide can also disrupt the body's acid-base balance, causing symptoms such as dizziness and lightheadedness. Furthermore, dysfunctional breathing can exacerbate existing respiratory conditions. For individuals with asthma, abnormal breathing patterns can trigger or worsen asthma symptoms, leading to increased wheezing, coughing, and breathlessness. Similarly, people with COPD may experience increased shortness of breath and reduced lung function due to dysfunctional breathing.

Managing dysfunctional breathing involves addressing both the physical and psychological aspects of the condition. Treatment approaches can vary depending on the underlying causes and severity of symptoms. Here are some common strategies:

1. Breathing retraining: Working with a healthcare professional, such as a respiratory therapist or physiotherapist, to learn proper breathing techniques. Techniques like diaphragmatic breathing paced breathing, and relaxation exercises can help restore a more balanced and efficient breathing pattern.

2. Physical activity and exercise: Engaging in regular physical activity can improve overall lung function and enhance respiratory muscle strength. Activities like yoga, tai chi, and swimming promote diaphragmatic breathing and relaxation.

3. Stress management: Since stress and anxiety contribute to dysfunctional breathing, learning stress management techniques like meditation, mindfulness, and deep relaxation can be beneficial. These practices help reduce the body's physiological response to stress and promote a more relaxed breathing pattern.

4. Posture correction: Maintaining good posture throughout the day supports optimal breathing mechanics. Being mindful of posture and avoiding slouching or hunching over ensures proper alignment of the diaphragm and facilitates efficient breathing.

5. Medications: In some cases, medication may be prescribed to manage underlying respiratory conditions or alleviate specific symptoms associated with dysfunctional breathing.

dysfunctional breathing is an abnormal or inefficient way of breathing that disrupts the natural breathing pattern. It can have physical and psychological symptoms, affect overall health, and worsen respiratory conditions. Managing dysfunctional breathing involves breathing retraining, physical activity, stress management, posture correction, and, if necessary, medication. By addressing both the physical and psychological aspects of the condition, individuals can restore a more balanced and efficient breathing pattern, leading to improved well-being and respiratory function

Chapter.7

Over-breathing

Over-breathing, also known as hyperventilation, refers to the condition where an individual engages in rapid or deep breathing that exceeds the body's oxygen demands. This common response can be triggered by various physical and emotional factors and has notable impacts on our overall well-being. Although occasional episodes of over-breathing may not cause significant harm, chronic or prolonged hyperventilation can lead to a range of symptoms and health issues.

When we breathe, we inhale oxygen and exhale carbon dioxide. Carbon dioxide is a waste product that accumulates in our bloodstream and needs to be expelled through exhalation. However, during over-breathing, excessive amounts of carbon dioxide are expelled, disrupting the delicate balance of gases in our bodies. Consequently, this can result in a range of physiological and psychological changes.

Dizziness or lightheadedness is one of the primary symptoms associated with over-breathing. This occurs because low levels of carbon dioxide can cause blood vessels in the brain to constrict, thereby reducing blood flow and oxygen delivery. Additionally, over-breathing can lead to the feeling of shortness of breath, as the body may perceive a lack of oxygen, even when actual oxygen levels are normal.

Tingling or numbness in the extremities, such as the hands, fingers, or feet, is another common symptom of over-breathing. This is caused by respiratory alkalosis, a condition that arises due to reduced carbon dioxide levels in the blood. Low carbon dioxide levels can affect the body's ability to release oxygen to the tissues, leading to altered sensations.

Chest pain or tightness can also be experienced as a result of over-breathing. Rapid breathing can cause the muscles around the chest and neck to become tense or constricted, resulting in discomfort. Additionally, over-breathing can trigger panic attacks or anxiety symptoms, as the rapid breathing pattern can activate the body's stress response and create a cycle of anxiety.

It's important to note that over-breathing can be both a cause and a consequence of anxiety or stress. Individuals who are already prone to anxiety may be more likely to engage in over-breathing as a response to stressors, which, in turn, can exacerbate their anxiety symptoms. Similarly, chronic over-breathing can perpetuate a cycle of anxiety and stress, making it challenging to break free from the pattern.

Addressing and managing over-breathing involves several approaches. First and foremost, awareness of the problem is crucial. Recognizing the symptoms and understanding the underlying causes can help individuals take proactive steps to reduce hyperventilation episodes. Breathing exercises, such as diaphragmatic breathing or pursed-lip breathing, can be beneficial in slowing down the breathing rate and restoring a more balanced pattern.

In some cases, medical intervention may be necessary, especially if over-breathing is associated with an underlying medical condition. For instance, individuals with respiratory disorders like asthma or chronic obstructive pulmonary disease (COPD) may require specific treatments or medications to manage their breathing patterns effectively.

Psychological interventions can also play a vital role in addressing over-breathing. Cognitive-behavioral therapy (CBT) is a commonly used approach that helps individuals identify and modify negative thoughts, emotions, and behaviors associated with hyperventilation. Relaxation techniques, such as progressive muscle relaxation or mindfulness meditation, can aid in reducing overall anxiety levels and promoting healthier breathing habits.

In conclusion, over-breathing or hyperventilation is a condition characterized by rapid or deep breathing that exceeds the body's oxygen demands. It can have significant effects on physical and mental well-being, leading to symptoms such as dizziness, shortness of breath, tingling or numbness, and chest pain. Managing over-breathing involves awareness, breathing exercises, medical intervention if necessary, and psychological approaches like CBT and

 relaxation techniques. By addressing this condition, individuals can regain control over their breathing patterns and improve their overall quality of life.

Chapter.8

Asthma

It affects millions of individuals worldwide and can range in severity from mild to severe, significantly impacting their quality of life.

The exact cause of asthma remains not fully elucidated, but it is believed to arise from a combination of genetic predisposition and environmental influences. Those with a family history of asthma or allergies are at a higher risk of developing the condition. Furthermore, exposure to allergens such as dust mites, pollen, pet dander, and mold can trigger asthma symptoms in susceptible individuals. Other triggers include respiratory infections, physical exertion, cold air, air pollution, and certain medications.

Airway inflammation is a key characteristic of asthma. Inflammation leads to redness, swelling, and increased sensitivity of the airways, making them more susceptible to narrowing and obstruction. When a person with asthma encounters a trigger, the muscles surrounding the airways contract, and excessive mucus production by the airway lining further impede airflow. These processes result in the hallmark symptoms of asthma, which can vary in intensity and duration.

Diagnosing asthma typically involves a comprehensive assessment of medical history, physical examination, and lung function tests. Healthcare professionals evaluate the frequency and severity of symptoms and assess the response to bronchodilator medications. Spirometry, a lung function test, is commonly employed to measure the forced exhalation of air after a deep breath. This test helps gauge the extent of airflow limitation and aids in determining the severity of asthma.

The treatment of asthma focuses on symptom control, prevention of exacerbations, and improvement of lung function. Asthma management follows a stepwise approach, with treatment intensity adjusted according to the severity of the condition. Bronchodilators, which relax the muscles of the airways, are the primary medications used. Short-acting bronchodilators provide quick relief during acute episodes, while long-acting bronchodilators are employed for long-term control. Inhaled corticosteroids are also frequently

prescribed to reduce airway inflammation and prevent exacerbations.
In addition to medication, individuals with asthma are often advised to identify and avoid triggers that can worsen their symptoms. This may involve making changes to the home environment, such as using dust mite-proof covers on mattresses and pillows, maintaining low indoor humidity levels, and regularly cleaning carpets and upholstery. Avoiding tobacco smoke, air pollution, and other irritants is also recommended.

Education and self-management play a crucial role in the care of asthma. Individuals with asthma should be knowledgeable about their condition, able to recognize early signs of worsening symptoms, and proficient in using their inhaler devices correctly. Asthma action plans, developed in collaboration with healthcare providers, provide guidelines on adjusting medication usage and when to seek medical assistance during exacerbations.
While asthma is a chronic condition, most individuals

with asthma are able to lead normal, active lives with proper management. However, severe asthma can be debilitating and may require additional
While asthma is a chronic condition, most individuals with asthma are able to lead normal, active lives with proper management. However, severe asthma can be debilitating and may require additional interventions, such as oral corticosteroids or biological therapies that target specific immune pathways involved in asthma inflammation.

Ongoing research in the field of asthma continues to enhance our understanding of the disease and improve treatment options. Scientists are investigating the underlying mechanisms of asthma, searching for new therapeutic targets, and exploring potential gene-environment interactions. This continuous research provides hope for the development of better asthma management strategies and novel treatments in the future.

 asthma is a chronic respiratory condition characterized by airway inflammation, bronchial hyperresponsiveness, and recurrent symptoms such as wheezing and shortness of breath. It affects millions of people worldwide and can significantly impact their daily lives. Through proper diagnosis, medication, trigger avoidance, education, and ongoing research, individuals with asthma can effectively manage their condition and lead fulfilling lives.

Chapter.9

Breathing disordered sleep

Breathing-disordered sleep, also known as sleep-disordered breathing (SDB), is a complex and prevalent health issue that affects a substantial portion of the population. It comprises a diverse spectrum of conditions characterized by disruptions in normal breathing patterns during sleep, giving rise to various symptoms and potential health consequences. While obstructive sleep apnea (OSA) is the most well-known form of breathing-disordered sleep, there are other conditions, including central sleep apnea and hypoventilation disorders, that fall within this category and warrant attention.

Obstructive sleep apnea is extensively studied and recognized as a prevalent form of breathing-disordered sleep. It occurs when the upper airway becomes partially or completely obstructed during sleep, leading to repetitive pauses in breathing known as apneas. These apneas can last for seconds to minutes and can occur multiple times throughout the night. As a result, sleep patterns are disrupted, and the delivery of oxygen to vital organs, including the brain, is compromised.

The primary risk factor for obstructive sleep apnea is obesity, as excess weight can contribute to the narrowing of the airway. However, other factors such as age, sex, anatomical abnormalities, and genetic predisposition can also play a role in its development. Common symptoms of obstructive sleep apnea include loud and chronic snoring, daytime sleepiness, morning headaches, difficulty concentrating, irritability, and waking up with a dry mouth or sore throat.

In contrast, central sleep apnea is caused by a failure of the brain to transmit appropriate signals to the muscles responsible for breathing. Consequently, individuals with central sleep apnea exhibit a lack of effort to breathe during sleep, resulting in breathing pauses. Unlike obstructive sleep apnea, the airway itself is not physically obstructed in central sleep apnea. Risk factors for this form of sleep-disordered breathing include certain medical conditions such as congestive heart failure, stroke, brainstem abnormalities, and the use of specific medications.

Hypoventilation disorders are characterized by inadequate ventilation during sleep, leading to elevated levels of carbon dioxide (hypercapnia) and reduced levels of oxygen (hypoxemia) in the blood. These disorders can be caused by conditions such as obesity hypoventilation syndrome (OHS), neuromuscular disorders, chest wall deformities, or respiratory muscle weakness. Symptoms may include daytime sleepiness, fatigue, morning headaches, and difficulty breathing.

Regardless of the specific condition, breathing-disordered sleep can have significant consequences for an individual's overall health and well-being. The repetitive disruptions in sleep patterns can lead to chronic sleep deprivation, resulting in daytime fatigue, impaired cognitive function, and decreased quality of life. Furthermore, untreated sleep-disordered breathing increases the risk of developing or exacerbating other medical conditions, including hypertension, cardiovascular disease, stroke, diabetes, and mood disorders.

Diagnosis of breathing-disordered sleep typically involves a comprehensive evaluation, including a thorough medical history assessment, physical examination, and sleep studies. Polysomnography, which monitors various physiological parameters during sleep, such as brain activity, eye movements, muscle tone, heart rate, and respiratory effort, is considered the gold standard for diagnosis.

Treatment options for breathing-disordered sleep vary depending on the specific condition and its severity. For obstructive sleep apnea, continuous positive airway pressure (CPAP) therapy is commonly prescribed. This therapy involves wearing a mask over the nose or mouth during sleep, which delivers a continuous flow of pressurized air to keep the airway open. Other treatment modalities include oral appliances that reposition the jaw and tongue, lifestyle modifications such as weight loss and avoiding alcohol or sedatives, and, in some cases, surgical interventions.

Central sleep apnea and hypoventilation disorders may require additional interventions, such as addressing the underlying medical conditions or using specialized breathing devices to assist with ventilation.

In conclusion, breathing-disordered sleep encompasses a wide range of conditions that can have a significant impact on an individual's health and well-being. Understanding the different forms of sleep-disordered breathing, their risk factors, symptoms, and potential consequences is crucial for timely diagnosis and appropriate management. By addressing breathing-disordered sleep, we can improve sleep quality, enhance overall health outcomes, and promote a better quality of life for affected individuals.

Chapter.10

Breathing with pain

Breathing is an innate and vital function of the human body, sustaining our existence without conscious effort. Unfortunately, we often take this automatic process for granted, only realizing its significance when pain disrupts our breathing patterns. The impact of pain on our physical and emotional well-being cannot be understated.

Pain is a complex sensation that can originate from various sources within our bodies. It may manifest as acute pain resulting from injuries or surgical procedures, or it can be chronic, stemming from conditions such as arthritis, fibromyalgia, or nerve damage. Irrespective of its origin, pain has the potential to affect every aspect of our lives, including the way we breathe.

When we experience pain, particularly in the chest or abdominal regions, our breathing tends to become shallow or restricted. There are several reasons behind this phenomenon. Firstly, pain itself can cause muscle tension and spasms, leading to a limited range of motion in the chest and abdomen. Consequently, the expansion and contraction of the lungs may be hindered, impeding the smooth flow of air and compromising the efficiency of breathing.

Furthermore, pain can trigger a physiological response known as the "fight-or-flight" response. This response activates the sympathetic nervous system, resulting in increased heart rate, elevated blood pressure, and shallow breathing. While these changes are intended to prepare the body for immediate action, they exacerbate the discomfort associated with pain, making breathing an even more challenging task.

The act of breathing in pain can also have a profound psychological impact. Chronic pain, in particular, has the potential to cause emotional distress, anxiety, and depression, further complicating our breathing patterns. The fear of experiencing pain with each breath can create a vicious cycle, where anxiety about breathing intensifies the pain, leading to increased anxiety, and so on.

Effectively managing breathing with pain requires a comprehensive approach that addresses both the physical and psychological aspects of the experience. Here are several strategies that can help individuals cope with pain while maintaining optimal breathing:

1. Relaxation techniques: Practices such as deep breathing exercises, progressive muscle relaxation, and meditation can help reduce muscle tension, promote relaxation, and improve breathing patterns.

2. Pain management techniques: Utilizing medications, physical therapy, heat or cold therapy, and other pain management strategies can help alleviate the underlying cause of the pain, making breathing more comfortable.

3. Breathing exercises: Techniques like diaphragmatic breathing, pursed-lip breathing, and paced breathing can enhance lung function, increase oxygenation, and reduce shortness of breath. These exercises focus on slowing down the breathing rate, prolonging exhalation, and engaging the diaphragm for more efficient breathing.

4. Positioning: Finding a comfortable position, such as sitting upright or propping oneself with pillows, can facilitate deeper breathing and alleviate discomfort.

5. Psychological support: Seeking emotional support from friends, family, or professionals such as therapists or support groups can help individuals navigate the psychological impact of living with pain. Techniques such as cognitive-behavioral therapy can assist in managing anxiety and depression associated with chronic pain.

6. Physical conditioning: Engaging in regular exercise, under the guidance of a healthcare professional, can strengthen the muscles involved in breathing and improve overall lung capacity. However, it is essential to find activities that are suitable for each individual's specific condition and pain tolerance.

7. Lifestyle modifications: Adopting a healthy lifestyle that includes a balanced diet, maintaining a healthy weight, getting enough sleep, and avoiding smoking can have a positive impact on pain management and overall well-being.

It is crucial to work closely with healthcare professionals to develop an individualized plan for managing pain and breathing difficulties. They can provide personalized guidance, recommend appropriate therapies, and monitor progress over time.

Breathing with pain can present significant challenges that affect various aspects of our lives. However, with the right approach, support, and strategies, individuals can find ways to cope, improve their breathing, and enhance their overall quality of life. By taking a comprehensive approach that addresses both the physical and psychological dimensions, individuals can regain control over their breathing, find relief from pain, and ultimately experience an improved sense of well-being.

Chapter.11

Breathing with anxiety

Understanding and effectively managing the physical and psychological symptoms of anxiety is crucial, and one area of utmost importance is breathing with anxiety. Anxiety is a prevalent mental health condition that affects millions of people worldwide, and it can manifest in various ways, including fear, restlessness, rapid heartbeat, and shortness of breath. These symptoms can be distressing and significantly interfere with daily life. However, one powerful tool for managing anxiety is conscious breathing.

When a person experiences anxiety, their body enters a state of heightened arousal known as the "fight-or-flight" response. This response triggers a series of physiological changes, including the release of stress hormones like adrenaline and cortisol. While these changes prepare the body to deal with a perceived threat, they can also lead to shallow, rapid breathing or even hyperventilation.

In the context of anxiety, breathing patterns can become irregular and disrupted, exacerbating the symptoms. This creates a cycle where the physical symptoms of anxiety, such as shortness of breath or dizziness, intensify the feeling of anxiety itself, resulting in a feedback loop of increased stress and further breathing difficulties.

However, by consciously focusing on breathing and implementing specific breathing techniques, individuals with anxiety can regain control over their breath and help alleviate some of the associated symptoms. Here are a few techniques that can be particularly beneficial:

1. Diaphragmatic Breathing: Also referred to as deep belly breathing or abdominal breathing, this technique involves breathing deeply into the diaphragm instead of shallowly into the chest. To practice diaphragmatic breathing, place one hand on your belly and the other on your chest. Inhale deeply through your nose, allowing your abdomen to rise as you fill your lungs with air. Exhale slowly through your mouth, feeling your belly fall. Repeat this process several times, focusing on the sensation of the breath entering and leaving your body.

2. Box Breathing: This technique follows a simple pattern of inhalation, holding the breath, exhalation, and holding again, each for an equal count of time. Visualize tracing a square or a box with your breath. Start by inhaling deeply through your nose for a count of four. Then hold your breath for a count of four. Exhale slowly through your mouth for a count of four, and hold your breath again for a count of four. Repeat this sequence several times, maintaining a steady rhythm.

3. 4-7-8 Breathing: Developed by Dr. Andrew Weil, this technique emphasizes extended exhalation, which can help activate the body's relaxation response. Begin by placing the tip of your tongue behind your upper front teeth. Breathe in quietly through your nose to a mental count of four. Hold your breath for a count of seven. Exhale forcefully through your mouth to a count of eight, producing a "whoosh" sound. Repeat this cycle three more times.

4. Mindfulness Breathing: Mindfulness meditation involves directing your complete attention to the present moment. By focusing on your breath and observing it without judgment, you can cultivate a sense of calm and reduce anxiety. Find a comfortable position, close your eyes, and take a few deep breaths. Then shift your focus to your breath, feeling the sensation of the air entering and leaving your nostrils or the rise and fall of your abdomen. Whenever your mind wanders, gently guide your attention back to your breath.

These breathing techniques serve as powerful tools to regulate the body's stress response, promote relaxation, and reduce anxiety symptoms. Regular practice can help individuals become more attuned to their breath and develop a greater sense of control over their physiological and emotional states.

It is important to note that while breathing exercises can be helpful, they may not be sufficient as the sole treatment for anxiety disorders. If you or someone you know

 is struggling with anxiety that significantly impacts daily life, it is advisable to seek professional help from a mental health provider. They can provide a comprehensive assessment and develop a personalized treatment plan that may include various therapeutic approaches in addition to breathing techniques.

breathing with anxiety is a vital aspect of managing and reducing the symptoms associated with anxiety. By incorporating conscious breathing techniques into daily life, individuals can regain a sense of control over their breath, alleviate physical symptoms, and promote a greater sense of calm and well-being. Remember to be patient and persistent in your practice, as the benefits of conscious breathing often accumulate over time, leading to improved overall mental and emotional health.

Chapter.12

Benefits of breathing through your nose

Breathing is an essential function that sustains life, and while most people instinctively breathe through their nose, it's important to recognize the numerous benefits associated with this natural mode of respiration. Nasal breathing, which involves inhaling and exhaling primarily through the nostrils, as opposed to the mouth, offers a wide range of advantages for overall health and well-being. Let's delve deeper into the benefits of nasal breathing and explore why it's worth prioritizing.

1. Efficient Oxygenation: The nasal passages are marvelously designed to optimize the intake of oxygen. Within the nostrils, specialized structures like turbinates and cilia act as gatekeepers, filtering, warming, and humidifying the incoming air. This intricate filtration process eliminates harmful particles, pathogens, and irritants, preventing them from reaching the delicate lung tissues. Moreover, the nasal cavity boasts a larger surface area compared to the mouth, allowing for enhanced oxygen absorption.

2. Nitric Oxide Production: Nasal breathing stimulates the production and release of a valuable gas called nitric oxide (NO), which is generated in the paranasal sinuses and nasal passages. Nitric oxide plays a crucial role in maintaining healthy blood vessels, regulating blood pressure, enhancing oxygen delivery, and promoting overall cardiovascular health. By breathing through your nose, you actively support the production of this beneficial gas and reap its manifold advantages.

3. Improved Lung Function: Nasal breathing encourages proper diaphragmatic breathing, also known as belly breathing. This technique engages the diaphragm, a large muscle beneath the lungs, which promotes deep and efficient inhalation. By employing diaphragmatic breathing, you maximize oxygen uptake and enhance lung capacity, leading to improved respiratory function and increased energy levels.

4. Enhanced Oxygen Exchange: The nasal cavity houses an intricate network of capillaries, tiny blood vessels that help warm the air and facilitate efficient oxygen exchange with the bloodstream. As air passes through the nasal passages, these capillaries enable the transfer of oxygen from the inhaled air to the body's cells and tissues, thereby supporting optimal function and overall vitality.

5. Proper Airway Moisture: Breathing through the mouth can lead to excessive evaporation of moisture from the respiratory tract, resulting in dryness and irritation. On the other hand, nasal breathing helps maintain the ideal moisture balance in the airways. The nasal passages humidify the inhaled air, preventing dryness and reducing the risk of respiratory issues such as bronchitis and asthma.

6. Enhanced Lung Protection: The nose serves as a natural defense mechanism, shielding the lungs against potentially harmful substances in the air. The fine hairs inside the nostrils, known as cilia, play a pivotal role in this protection by trapping dust, allergens, and other airborne particles, preventing them from reaching the lungs. This inherent safeguard minimizes the risk of respiratory infections, allergies, and other respiratory disorders.

7. Improved Sleep Quality: Nasal breathing is particularly advantageous during sleep. By breathing through the nose, you help maintain an open airway, reducing the likelihood of snoring, sleep apnea, and other sleep-related breathing issues. Nasal breathing promotes a more relaxed state, enhances oxygen supply to the brain, and encourages deeper, more restful sleep.

8. Increased Mindfulness and Relaxation: Nasal breathing constitutes a fundamental component of various mindfulness and relaxation techniques, such as yoga and meditation. The deliberate focus on slow, conscious breaths through the nose aids in calming the mind, reducing stress, and inducing a state of relaxation. Nasal breathing cultivates present-moment awareness, supporting mental clarity and emotional balance.

breathing through your nose offers a multitude of benefits for your overall health and well-being. From efficient oxygenation and improved lung function to enhanced lung protection and better sleep quality, nasal breathing plays a crucial role in optimizing respiratory health. By prioritizing nasal breathing and practicing conscious breathwork, you can harness the power of this natural physiological process to enhance your vitality, reduce the risk of respiratory issues, and promote a sense of calm and well-being.

Chapter.13

Buteyko breathing education exercises

Buteyko breathing education exercises were originally developed in the 1950s by Dr. Konstantin Buteyko, a Russian physician, and have since gained recognition as a valuable tool for improving respiratory health and overall well-being. By focusing on reducing breathing rates and restoring the body's natural balance of oxygen and carbon dioxide, these exercises offer a holistic approach to enhancing one's respiratory function.

At the core of Buteyko breathing lies the understanding that many individuals tend to over breathe or hyperventilate, leading to a decrease in carbon dioxide levels in the body. This disruption of the optimal balance of gases in the blood can have various negative effects on health. The primary goal of Buteyko exercises is to retrain the breath and diminish excessive breathing.

The exercises encompass a range of techniques and lifestyle adjustments that address hyperventilation. Nasal breathing takes center stage in Buteyko exercises, requiring individuals to consciously inhale and exhale through the nose rather than the mouth. This practice aids in filtering, warming, and humidifying the air, thus promoting optimal respiratory function. Another technique involves breath holds, where individuals hold their breath for a short period after exhaling, effectively increasing carbon dioxide levels in the blood.

Buteyko breathing exercises have proven beneficial in managing various respiratory conditions, including asthma, chronic obstructive pulmonary disease (COPD), and anxiety-related breathing disorders. Studies have indicated that these exercises can alleviate symptoms, improve lung function, and potentially reduce the reliance on medication for some individuals. Moreover, they have been recognized for their potential to reduce stress, enhance sleep quality, and boost athletic performance.

It is essential to approach Buteyko breathing exercises with proper guidance from a qualified instructor. These exercises are tailored to each individual's specific needs and may require adjustments based on their health condition and fitness level. By receiving proper instruction and engaging in regular practice, individuals can maximize the benefits of Buteyko breathing and develop healthier breathing patterns that contribute to improved overall well-being.

some commonly used Buteyko breathing exercises:

Buteyko breathing exercises encompass a range of techniques that can be beneficial for improving respiratory function and overall well-being. By incorporating these exercises into your daily routine, you can experience the following benefits:

1. Nasal Breathing: One of the fundamental practices in Buteyko breathing is consciously breathing through the nose instead of the mouth. By doing so, you allow the air to be filtered, humidified and warmed before it reaches your lungs. Nasal breathing promotes optimal oxygen uptake and helps maintain the ideal moisture levels in your respiratory system.

2. Reduced Breathing: This exercise focuses on reducing the volume of air taken in with each breath. It involves gentle and slow breathing, emphasizing a relaxed exhale. The key is to avoid deep or forceful inhalations. By breathing less air, you can maintain a state of calm and relaxation while still meeting your body's oxygen needs.

3. Breath Holds: Breath holds are designed to increase the levels of carbon dioxide in your blood and improve your tolerance to higher carbon dioxide levels. After a gentle exhale, you briefly pause before taking your next inhalation. Over time, you can gradually increase the duration of these breath holds as your tolerance improves.

4. Control Pause: The control pause is a measure of your breath-holding time and is used as a baseline to track your progress. To determine your control pause, take a normal breath in and out, and then hold your breath until you feel the first natural urge to breathe again. The duration of this breath hold is noted and can be compared over time to assess improvements in your respiratory function.

5. Relaxation Techniques: Buteyko exercises often incorporate relaxation techniques such as progressive muscle relaxation, meditation, and mindfulness. These techniques help reduce stress and tension in the body, allowing for a more natural and efficient breathing pattern. By incorporating these relaxation techniques, you can further enhance the benefits of the breathing exercises.

6. Physical Activity with Nasal Breathing: Engaging in physical activity while practicing nasal breathing can be challenging but highly beneficial. By gradually increasing the intensity of your exercise while maintaining nasal breathing, you can enhance your respiratory fitness and adapt to a more efficient breathing pattern. This practice can improve your overall athletic performance and endurance.

It's important to note that consistent practice and patience are key to experiencing the full benefits of Buteyko breathing techniques. Incorporating these exercises into your daily routine and maintaining regular practice will help you develop a healthier and more efficient breathing pattern, leading to improved respiratory function and overall well-being.

Some of the qualities of breath

The qualities of breath hold profound insights into our physical, mental, and emotional well-being, offering a glimpse into the very essence of life itself. Across various cultures and spiritual traditions, breath is recognized as a vital force that connects us to the core of our existence. In this exploration, we delve into the qualities of breath and delve deeper into their significance, unlocking the power they hold.

1. Rhythm: At its core, breath embodies a rhythmic essence. Its cyclical pattern of inhalation and exhalation mirrors the natural rhythms found in the universe—the rising and setting of the sun, the ebb, and flow of the tides. By attuning ourselves to the rhythm of our breath, we align with these larger cosmic patterns, discovering a sense of harmony and equilibrium within.

2. Depth: The depth of our breath refers to the extent to which we fill our lungs during inhalation. Shallow breaths are typically swift and limited to the chest, while deep breaths are slower and expand into the abdomen. Deep breathing is closely linked to relaxation, stress reduction, and optimal oxygenation of the body. Through purposefully deepening our breath, we activate the body's relaxation response, fostering a profound sense of tranquility and well-being.

3. Awareness: The quality of awareness in our breath revolves around being fully present and attentive to the act of breathing. Our minds often wander, detaching from the breath as we become entangled in thoughts, concerns, and distractions. Nurturing awareness in our breath involves gently redirecting our attention back to the breath whenever we notice our minds wandering. This practice enriches mindfulness, forging a deeper connection with the present moment.

4. Smoothness: The smoothness of breath signifies a state devoid of strain, jerkiness, or irregularities in its flow. Smooth breathing reflects a relaxed state of being, where the breath moves effortlessly without any sense of force or obstruction. Stress, anxiety, or physical tension can disrupt the smoothness of our breath, causing it to become fragmented or constricted. By consciously striving for smooth breaths, we release tension, restore balance, and invite a sense of ease into our being.

5. Length: The length of our breath pertains to the duration of inhalation and exhalation. It varies depending on our emotional state, physical activity, and overall well-being. During moments of calm and relaxation, our breath naturally lengthens and slows down. Conversely, when we experience fear, anger, or excitement, our breath tends to become short and rapid. By intentionally elongating our breath, we activate the body's relaxation response, mitigating stress and fostering mental clarity.

6. Pause: Within the ebb and flow of breath lies the pause—a moment of stillness, a gap in which we can experience spaciousness and tranquility. Attending to these pauses assists in cultivating a deeper awareness of the present moment, fostering a state of calm and clarity within ourselves.

7. Synchronicity: The quality of synchronicity in breath refers to the alignment and coordination between breath and other bodily functions. Engaging in physical activities such as yoga, exercise, or meditation entails synchronizing our breath with our movements, enhancing focus, concentration, and energy flow. This synchronization fosters unity within ourselves, harmoniously connecting mind, body, and breath.

The qualities of breath unveil invaluable insights into our overall well-being, offering potent tools for self-regulation and personal growth. By developing an awareness of our breath and consciously cultivating its qualities, we tap into its potential to promote relaxation, reduce stress, enhance mental clarity, and forge a deeper connection with ourselves and the world around us. Breath emerges as a profound source of wisdom, an unwavering ally on our journey toward improved health, harmony, and self-discovery.

Conclusion

In conclusion, the concept of "inhaling freedom" presents an intriguing and forward-thinking approach to enhancing human comfort and well-being. By integrating breathable materials and technologies into various facets of our lives, ranging from clothing and accessories to architecture and transportation, we can forge a more breathable environment that promotes both physical and mental health.

The inhaling freedom concept acknowledges the significance of air circulation and the exchange of gases between our bodies and the surrounding environment. It recognizes that excessive heat and moisture buildup can detrimentally impact our comfort, productivity, and overall health. By prioritizing breathability, we have the opportunity to create spaces and products that optimize airflow, regulate temperature, and mitigate the risks associated with moisture, such as bacterial growth and unpleasant odors.

In the realm of fashion and clothing, the inhaling freedom concept holds immense potential. Breathable fabrics that facilitate the passage of air while still possessing crucial properties such as durability and protection have the power to revolutionize our approach to dressing. Such materials can keep us cool and dry, particularly in hot and humid climates, and alleviate discomfort and skin-related issues caused by trapped moisture.

Furthermore, the inhaling freedom concept extends beyond clothing and permeates other areas of our lives. In architecture and interior design, the integration of breathable materials and ventilation systems can greatly enhance indoor air quality, reduce the dependence on artificial cooling and heating, and establish more comfortable living and working environments. Similarly, in transportation, the incorporation of breathable materials can improve the air quality within vehicles, making travel more pleasant and healthier.

Embracing the inhaling freedom concept aligns seamlessly with our growing focus on sustainability and eco-consciousness. By facilitating better airflow and diminishing the need for energy-intensive climate control systems, breathable materials contribute to more energy-efficient and environmentally friendly practices.

However, while the potential benefits of the inhaling freedom concept are evident, further research and development are necessary. Innovations in material science, engineering, and design will play pivotal roles in advancing breathability and ensuring its practicality, versatility, and durability. Additionally, it is essential to consider the maintenance of appropriate levels of privacy and protection in various applications of breathability.

the inhaling freedom concept represents a promising approach to improving human comfort, health, and sustainability. By placing an emphasis on breathability in our clothing, architecture, and transportation, we can cultivate a more harmonious relationship between our bodies and the environment. Through continuous exploration and refinement, the inhaling freedom concept has the potential to transform the way we live, work, and interact with the world around us.